HISTOLOGY

2017/18

COURSE INFORMATION

AND

LECTURE NOTES

JF Medicine
JF Physiotherapy

Dr Alan R Tuffery

Department of Physiology

Illustrations with the assistance of Mr Quentin Comerford
and Mr Aidan Kelly

CONTENTS

INTRODUCTION

Histology is the study of tissue structure, extending from the level of the individual cell, through organs to organ systems. Histology is obviously related to *Cell Biology (Cytology)* and to *Anatomy*; it also forms the structural basis for understanding Function (*Physiology*) and is the preparation for the study of abnormal structure and function (*Pathology*). Pathophysiological (clinical) examples will be used to illustrate aspects of functions and their significance.

The principal aim of the course is to provide a knowledge of tissue structure which is sufficient for the understanding of Physiology.

Tissues may be regarded as aggregations of cells (of one, or more usually, several types) which serve a particular function or set of functions.

From this definition it will be seen that the concepts of structure and function are essential to the study of Histology

Particular *skills which* will be emphasised are:

a) *Classification* of tissues — essentially a *verbal skill*. Consequently it is important to pay close attention to the way tissues are described. This means concentrating on the precise and correct use of language — an essential skill in sciences, and the health-care professions.

b) *Recognition* of specific features and the application of the criteria of classification — *observational and reasoning skills*.

c) Most importantly, the *relationship between structure and function*. This means bringing together knowledge from different fields (e.g. Anatomy, Biochemistry and Physiology) — *synthetic* and *deductive* skills.

Assumed background knowledge

a) Basic cell structure, including electron microscopy and cell organelles.

b) Methods of tissue preparation: fixing, sectioning and staining.

Both of these topics should be rapidly revised by reading the first one or two chapters of almost any Histology textbook (see page 2 ff for notes on recommended textbooks).

It is important to know how the method of preparation affects the tissue. In particular, the effects of making a virtually two-dimensional section of a three-dimensional structure must always be taken into account. The functional state of the tissue should also be taken into account: a histological preparation is a *static* representation of a *dynamic* process.

Biology

Students who have not previously studied Biology should make a special effort to get a basic grounding from a Leaving Certificate or JF Biology text as soon as possible. The key areas are cell structure and function and the basic functions of the organs of the body. The JF Biology text is Biology by Campbell, NA & Reece, JB. There are multiple copies of the 6th *edition (2002) in the Hamilton reserve collection (shelf mark 574 M84*5;35).*

Lecture Synopses

Synopses of lectures are provided to give the basic minimum information for this course. They should be read *before* the corresponding lecture in order to minimise the amount of note-taking and thereby leave you free to study the *images*, concentrate on the *language* used and focus on the *key concepts*.

The terminology used in the lectures and summaries is that agreed by international convention, as set out in *Nomina Histologica* (1975), and will sometimes differ from that in textbooks. The most important difference is the deletion of all eponymous terms (i.e. those bearing individuals' names). The modern terminology tends to be usefully descriptive (e.g. 'intestinal crypts' for 'crypts of Lieberkühn').

The course manual includes *learning outcomes* for each week of the course.

Supports

Students who need additional supports because of a disability should arrange to discuss their position with Dr Tuffery Contact Person for Disability Support in the Department of Physiology.

This manual is available in electronic (PDF) format from my Get folder on the ISS system or in large print from Dr Alan Lecture slides are available — usually before each lecture — from my GET folder. Podcasts may be available.

STRUCTURE OF THE COURSE

In Michaelmas Term the course deals with *Basic Tissues, Body Fluids* and *Blood* (including basic immunology etc).

    i)   *Lectures.* There are seven Lectures (See *Course Handbook*).
    ii)   *Practical Classes.* There are two practical classes per student.

        a)   Medical students have a two practical classes in the Biology Laboratory, East End
        b)   *Computer-Aided Instruction.* A suite of images and related MCQs is available private study on College's public access computers at http://www.tcd.ie/Physiology/text/software/download.html.

ASSESSMENT

Questions on this part of the course will appear in the integrated examinations of the year (see *Course Handbook*).

Outline of Lectures

Lecture I *Introduction*
General — synopses, organisation of course
Classification of tissues: the four Basic Tissues (Epithelium, Connective Tissue, Muscle and Nerve)
Function and features of epithelia — permeability/transport
Classification of epithelia
Cell surface specialisation and functions

Lecture 2 *Connective Tissue Proper*
Functional significance: 'support'
Components *(selected* cell types, fibres, matrix)
Examples (incl. areolar, adipose [BAT, WAT])
Interrelationship of CT cell types (incl. Blood)
Cartilage (incl. growth).

Lecture 3 *Excitable Tissues*
Muscle: Smooth, cardiac, skeletal; appearance, function innervation The motor unit
Nerve: fibres, cells, synapse
Skeletal muscle-fibre types

Lecture 4 *Bone*
Structure of Bone (gross, histology, components)
Bone formation (intracartilaginous ossification) as a process:-
growth, destruction of cartilage, ossification, remodelling
Bone dynamics — osteoblasts and osteoclasts; regulation of Ca^{2+}

Lecture 5 *Body Fluids*
Fluid compartments — definition and volumes
Movement of fluid between compartments (oedema) — significance
Differences in composition
Inputs and outputs
Regulation of composition of Plasma — significance

Lecture 6 *Blood*
Haematocrit
Plasma proteins
Importance of recognition of circulating cells
Functions
Clotting
Formation (haemopoiesis)
Fundamentals of anaemias

Lecture 7 *Immunology*
Components
Innate and Adaptive Immunity
Immune disorders

DESCRIPTION OF CELLS AND TISSUES

An essential requirement in Histology is to be able to describe cells and tissues unambiguously. The following list gives all the criteria which can be used at light microscope level.

a) *Relative size* — e.g. compared to other cells in the tissue.

b) *Shape* — e.g. columnar, cuboidal, flattened, polyhedral.

c) *Cytoplasmic reaction* usually refers to acidophilia (usually eosinophilia, i.e. affinity for eosin) or basophilia (usually affinity for haematoxylin), although special stains may be used for specific substances (e.g. fat or glycogen).

e) *Cytoplasmic inclusions* — e.g. granules, vacuoles.

e) *Nuclear characteristics* — e.g. shape, position within the cell, size, staining pattern, presence or absence of nucleoli.

f) *Surface specialisations* — e.g. cilia.

g) *Arrangement* — cells are arranged to form tissues, e.g. in single or multiple layers, cords or clumps; with variable amounts of intercellular matrix which may be solid, fluid or fibrous.

— — — — — —

HAEMATOXYLIN & EOSIN STAINING

Haematoxylin and eosin (usually abbreviated H&E) are two very commonly used histological stains. It is most important to be clear about their properties because the interpretation of cell function depends upon a knowledge of the reaction (pH) of organelles.

Haematoxylin is a base and therefore tends to bind to acidic structures. It stains blue. The most distinctive acid in cells is nuclear DNA, consequently nuclei appear blue. Structures which are acidic are said to be *basophilic*, i.e. they attract basic stains.

Eosin is acidic and therefore stains basic structures. It stains red. The cytoplasm of most cells is slightly basic and therefore stains pink and is said to be *acidophilic*.

Note that a knowledge of these properties allows you to interpret a preparation made with an unknown stain. The nucleus is always acidic and therefore defines the *basic* stain.

BASIC TISSUES

Classically, the Basic Tissues are: *Epithelia*, *Connective Tissue* and the *Excitable Tissues* (Nerve and Muscle). This is a core concept of this course.

EPITHELIAL TISSUES

Objectives

a) To be able to list the Basic Tissues and their general functions
b) To be able to state the general function of lining epithelia.
c) To be able to classify lining epithelia according to morphological criteria.
d) To be able to relate structure and function in lining epithelia
e) To be able to give examples of named epithelia: structure, location, function.

––––––––

[*Epithelium* — a single tissue; plural, *epithelia*; adjective, *epithelial*]

There are two functional types of epithelium: lining epithelia and glandular epithelium.

Lining Epithelia — cover the free surfaces of the body and its cavities, e.g. epidermis, lining of the gastrointestinal tract and ducts.

Their position in contact with the environment gives them great importance in regulating the composition of the body by controlling the movement of materials in and out.

The structure of lining epithelia can be correlated with their function. Thus the epithelium of larger ducts is thicker than in smaller ducts; and in sites exposed to desiccation or friction the epithelium may have a surface coat of keratin, a tough protein, and is said to be *keratinised*. (For specific examples of the adaptation of epithelia to particular function see the organ systems.)

Many epithelia have a high rate of renewal of their constituent cells. For example, the entire epithelium of the gut is replaced every 6-7 days (equivalent to a daily loss of $1.38 \times 10_9$ cells from the small intestine).

1. Structural Characterisation of Epithelia

a) *absence of nerves* (except for a few axons in the deeper layers)
b) *absence of blood vessels* — nutrition is by diffusion from the highly vascular connective tissue (known as the *lamina propria*) underlying all epithelia
c) *close packing* of the constituent cells with minimal intercellular substance.

2. Morphological Classification of Epithelia (Figure 1)

a) **number of layers of cells**: an epithelium with only one layer is described as *simple*; with more layers — *stratified*. (Note that *cells* are not described as 'simple' or 'stratified', only the *layer*.)

N.B. *Pseudostratified epithelium* appears to be more than one cell thick since the nuclei lie at different heights, but in fact all cells are in contact with the basement membrane (see Figure 1d).

b) **shape of cells at *free surface*:** e.g. *squamous* (flattened), *cuboidal*, *columnar*.

c) **surface specialisation** (if any) e.g. *keratinised*, *ciliated*.

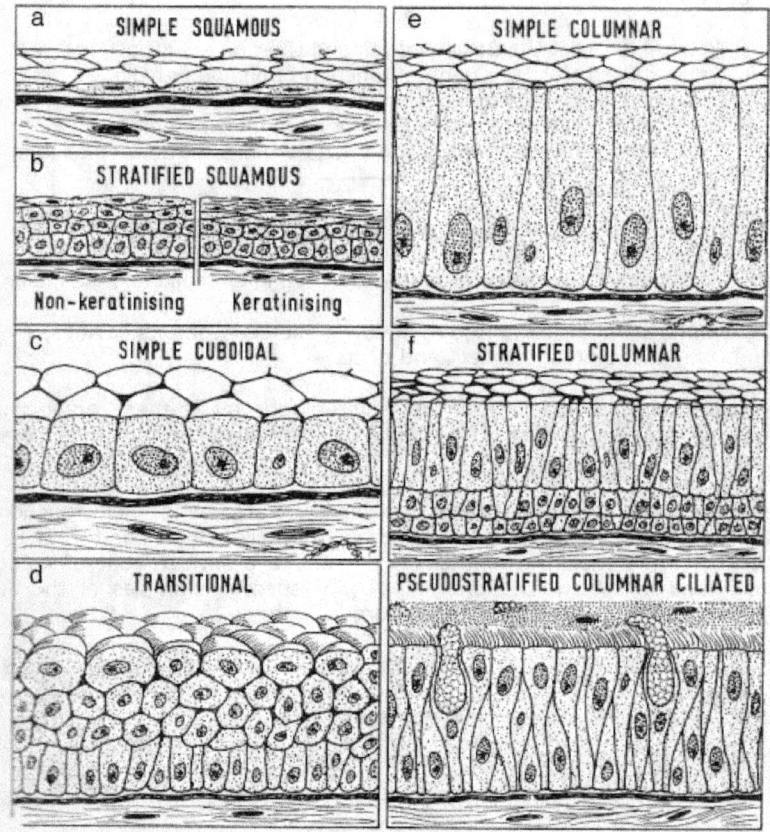

Figure 1 Diagram of types of lining epithelium

a) *Simple squamous epithelium* — a single layer of flattened cells. *Function*. The thinness provides minimal barrier to the movement of materials.

Examples. Alveolar lining of the lung, renal corpuscle.

b) *Simple cuboidal epithelium* — a single layer of box-shaped (cuboidal) cells. *Function*. Usually have a role in active transport or synthesis. *Examples*. Lining of ducts, thyroid follicles.

c) *Simple columnar epithelium* — a single layer of tall cells.
    Function. Metabolically active cells — absorption, synthesis.
    Example. Lining of intestine.

d) *Pseudostratified columnar ciliated epithelium* — although nuclei lie at different levels, all the cells are attached to the basement membrane and so there is only one layer.
    Function. Complex — several different functions.
    Example. Lining of trachea.

e) *Transitional epithelium* — there are several layers of cells; those at the free or luminal surface are irregularly polyhedral (like squashed bubbles) and it is called transitional.
    Function. To allow large changes in the volume of the lumen.
    Examples. Bladder, ureter.

f) *Stratified squamous epithelium* — Many layers of cells; those at the free surface are flattened.
    Function. To withstand mechanical wear and tear; resist desiccation *Example*. Lining of mouth, vagina and rectum.

g) *Stratified squamous epithelium (keratinised)* — the surface cells are dead and filled with an inert protein, keratin, forming flakes or *squames*.
    Function. As (f), but more so.
    Example. Skin.

——————

Test Questions on Epithelia

1. List the three criteria used to classify lining epithelia.

2. Give a brief description of the terms used to describe the shape of the surface cells in lining epithelia.

3. List two types of surface specialisation found in lining epithelia.

[Answers at end of text]

LECTURE 2

CONNECTIVE TISSUES

[Note — Wheater prefers the term 'supporting tissues' to reflect the wide range of important functions, but this is not yet generally accepted.]

Objectives

a) To be able to state the general functions of connective tissues.
b) To be able to state the names and properties of the principal fibre and cell types of CT.
c) To be able to outline the role of the matrix in conferring differing properties of CT.
d) To be able to give the basis of the morphological classification of CT.
e) To be able to relate structure to function of the different types of CT.
f) To recognise the inter-relatedness of all CT cells.

———————

Connective tissue (CT) occurs everywhere in the body in a variety of forms. Its principal function is support, both structural and physiological. It is both a skeletal framework for tissues and also the route through which blood vessels and nerves run. CT binds organs as in fascia and capsules of organs, and supports the other components of organs e.g. interlobular CT of glands and the *lamina propria* of epithelia. CT has an important function in modulating the differentiation and division of the overlying cells.

Histologically, CT is characterised by having cells scattered within varying amounts of extracellular material, which consists of fibres and ground substance (matrix).

1. Components of Connective Tissues

a) *Fibres* — collagenous, reticular or elastic.

b) *Cells* — of many types, including white blood cells which have left the blood vessels. Macrophages and fibroblasts are the commonest cell types. The cells are derived from a common precursor (ancestral) cell which is closely related to the precursor of blood cells. (See Figure 2.)

d) *Ground substance* — typically amorphous, may be sol/gel and is mainly composed of hyaluronic acid and glycoproteins (especially chondroitin sulphate). To a very large extent it is the properties of the different glycoproteins which determine the different properties of connective tissues. The types and arrangement of the glycoproteins varies within connective tissues and according to age.

In addition to *Connective Tissue Proper* there are the *Specialised Connective Tissues:* Blood, Cartilage, Bone and the Lymphoid organs (see below).

2. Classification of Connective Tissue Proper

a) **Proportion of fibres** (low — *Loose*; high — *Dense*). In practice, there is a graded series of density.

b) **Arrangement of fibres** — *Regular* (in parallel bundles) or *Irregular* (in a coarse feltwork).

3. Types of Connective Tissue Proper

3.1 Loose Connective Tissues

a) *Loose (Areolar) Connective Tissue.* Develops from mesenchyme. It occurs as packing and support of most structures (e.g. lamina propria underlying epithelia). Has all types of fibre with collagen the most conspicuous. Reticular fibres may be abundant at the edges of other structures. The unstained ground-substance occurs in patches (*areolae*).

Areolar CT is well-supplied with nerves and blood vessels which supply the overlying epithelium. Macrophages and fibroblasts are the predominant cell types.

c) *White Adipose Tissue* (WAT). Fat cells are the main cell type and are surrounded by reticular fibres. Because fat is dissolved out in by the alcohols used in histological preparation, the cells normally appear empty with a thin ring of cytoplasm. Note that *Brown Adipose Tissue* (BAT) has many small lipid droplets, in contrast to the single droplet in WAT. Adipose tissue is highly vascular reflecting the dynamic state of rapid metabolism and turnover of lipid.

e) *Reticular tissue.* 'Primitive', composed of probably pluripotent cells and reticular fibres. Found only in lymphoid tissues.

Other principal cell types: lymphoid cells, eosinophils and mast cells.

3.2 Dense Connective Tissues

Characterised by having a relatively high proportion of fibres.

a) *Dense Irregular Connective Tissue.* A coarse feltwork of mainly collagenous fibres forming sheets. Designed to withstand multidirectional stress.

b) *Dense Regular Connective Tissue.* Parallel fibres to withstand unidirectional stress. Fibroblasts are the predominant cell type. The predominant fibre type is collagen, except in special elastic ligaments.
Examples. Tendons and ligaments, where the collagen fibres are arranged into bundles or *fascicles*.

c) *Fibrocartilage*. Note that at the insertion of tendon on the surface of bone, Dense Regular CT blends into the cartilage. Thus, at this zone of transition there is a gradation from dense fibrous tissue of the tendon through calcified fibrocartilage to bone. The amount of fibrocartilage may vary in specific sites according to the differing stresses. For example, the lateral menisci of the knee-joint have more fibrocartilage than the medial because there is more movement in the former.

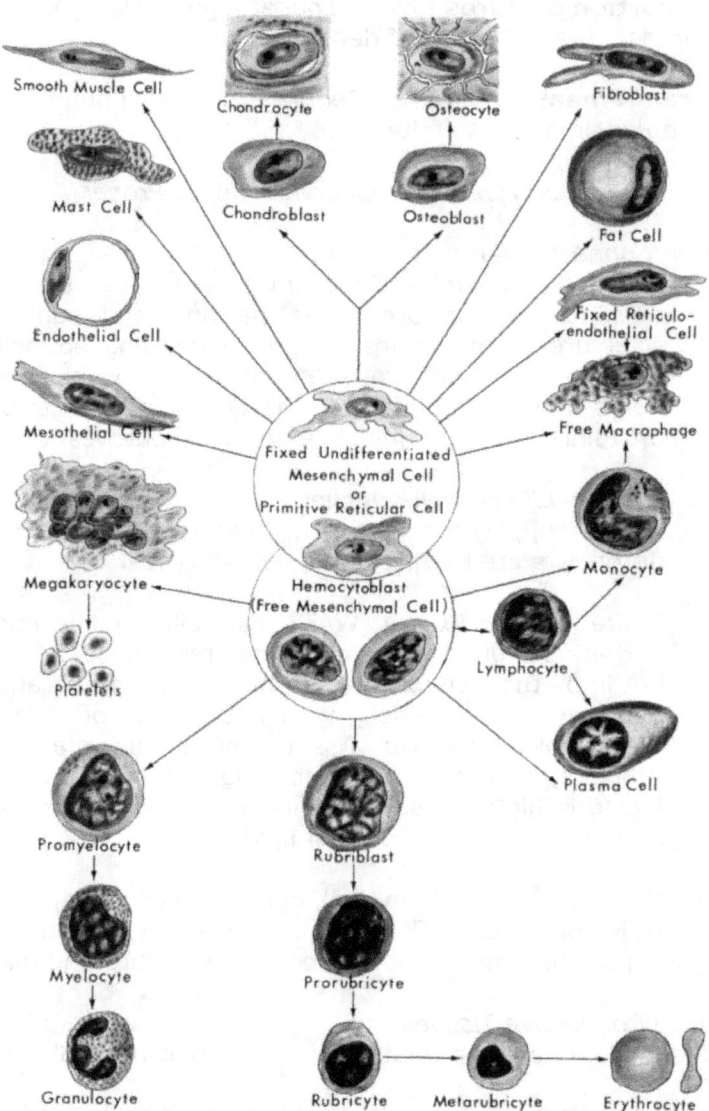

Figure 2. Relationship of connective tissue cell type and blood cells. The upper half of the figure shows the various types of connective tissue cells and emphasises their inter-relatedness. They all arise from one single precursor cell. The lower part of the figure shows the blood cells which arise from a single precursor cell which is closely related to the precursor cell of the other connective tissue. The lineage of the developing blood cells is shown in abbreviated form. *[From Leeson & Leeson 3rd edn]*

Test Questions on Connective Tissue Proper

1. What are the components of Connective Tissues?

2. What criteria are used to classify Connective Tissue Proper?

3. White Adipose Tissue is pale in a conventional, wax-embedded preparation because [Choose one answer]:
    a) fat is dissolved out in fixing
    b) fat is dissolved out in dehydration
    c) fat is dissolved out in staining
    d) fat stains only very lightly
    e) fat doesn't stain

4. How can fat be preserved in a slide?

[Answers at end of text]

————

4. Specialised Connective Tissues

These include *Cartilage*, *Bone* and *Blood*; and since cartilage precedes bone in development, the process of *Ossification* will be outlined (*Lecture 4*).

All three of the specialised CTs differ from *CT Proper* in that they have a greater proportion of extracellular matrix; in cartilage and bone the matrix is solid.

4.1 Cartilage
Develops from mesenchyme. Provides good support while retaining flexibility. Uniquely among connective tissues, it lacks blood vessels and nerves. There are three types of cartilage.

a) *Hyaline Cartilage*. The commonest type of cartilage. Cartilage cells (*chondrocytes*) occupy spaces (*lacunae*; singular, *lacuna*) in the matrix which is slightly basophilic due to high content of glycoproteins. The chondrocytes shrink in preparation and are vacuolated (due to the presence of unstained glycogen and lipid). Collagen fibres form a fine feltwork but are not visible with normal staining methods.
    Locations — larynx, trachea, bronchi, articular surfaces of joints.

b) *Elastic Cartilage* contains a large proportion of elastic fibres (demonstrable by special staining methods) for greater flexibility.
    Location — external ear.

c) *Fibrocartilage*. (See above, Section 3.2c) *Location*
    — tendinous insertions; vertebral disc.

LECTURE 3

EXCITABLE TISSUES

Objectives

    a) To be able to describe the structure and function of the different types of muscle.
    b) To be able to comment on their appearance in section.
    c) To describe the fibre-types of skeletal muscle.
    d) To be able to define a motor unit.
    e) To be able to describe the structure (whole and in section) and function of a neurone.
    f) To be able to describe myelinated and nonmyelinated nerve axons.

Muscle & Nerve: together the *Excitable Tissues*, characterised by response to external stimuli; part of response is electrical.

MUSCLE

Muscle is adapted for contraction. There are three types of muscle: *smooth*, *cardiac* and *skeletal*. They can be considered as a series of increasing specialisation for contraction.

Smooth Muscle

Consists of small spindle-shaped cells with central nuclei; the cells are not striated. Arranged in sheets or bundles (e.g. gut).

> *Innervation* — complex. *Dual* innervation with both excitatory and inhibitory inputs. The balance between them gives rise to a partial state of contraction or *tone*.
> In *single-unit* muscle (e.g. gut, uterus) not all cells are directly innervated; instead they are coupled more or less indirectly, so that excitation spreads from the directly-innervated cells to those that do not receive innervation. In *multi-unit* muscle (e.g. airways, large arteries) each cell is innervated.

> *Function*. Relatively weak slow, spreading contraction (obviously related to the above properties. The contraction of each cell is *graded* (cf. 'all-or none' of cardiac /skeletal muscle).

Cardiac Muscle

Consists of large cells or fibres joined end-to-end at intercalated discs (modified Z discs). The fibres are striated indicating an elaborate contractile apparatus. Fibres may branch and have electrical continuity; may be binucleate. Nuclei are central.

    Innervation. Within the heart pacemakers control the rate of contraction and excitation spreads via the left and right branch bundles of Purkinje fibres: modified cardiac muscle cells containing glycogen.

    Function — non-fatiguing, powerful, co-ordinated contraction; rich in mitochondria; rich blood supply.

Skeletal Muscle

The most highly specialised for contraction. Consists of large fibres: multinucleate with relatively prominent cross-striations

Innervation. Each fibre receives a single axon of an alpha motor neurone forming an endplate; a specialised form of neuromuscular junction, characterised by much folding of the post-synaptic (muscle) surface to give a large surface area for transmission.

One spinal motor neurone can innervate 100s of muscle fibres — *the motor unit.* There are many motor units in a muscle. Hence increasing power due to 'recruitment'.

Function. Fast, powerful, 'all or nothing' ('twitch') contraction.

Muscle Fibre-Types. Two main types of skeletal muscle fibre are recognised with varying physiological properties according to enzyme profiles. The principal enzymes used are succinic dehydrogenase (SDH), a mitochondrial oxidative enzyme and myofibrillar ATPase (mATPase). The Table below summarises the enzyme and physiological differences between Type I and Type II fibres. The fibre-type is determined largely by the neurone innervating it. The constituent fibres of a motor unit are scattered throughout a muscle ('mosaic' not 'random'). The property of an anatomical muscle depends upon the proportions of I and II.

Table. Some Properties of Types I and II Muscle Fibres

Enzyme activity	Type I	Type II
mATPase activity (anaerobic)	low	high
Oxidative capacity (aerobic)	high	low
Speed of contraction	slow	fast

NERVE

Adapted to the conduction of electrical impulses (action potentials). Transmission between one nerve terminal and another or an end-organ is by chemical transmission across the synaptic gap.

It is important to distinguish between anatomical nerves (with names); small nerves and nerve bundles (no names); nerve cell bodies; and nerve processes (nerve fibres, axons, dendrites).

Nerve Cells (neurones). Often only the 'cell body' is seen in section. Typically they are relatively large cells with a large pale nucleus with a prominent nucleolus. The cytoplasm contains many granules which are clusters of free ribosomes (the high RNA content makes them basophilic).

A typical motor neurone receives about 1000 connections, reflecting the general function of neurones of integrating inputs and giving a single output, the *action potential*. A neurone's connections may be relatively short and non-myelinated ('dendrites') or longer (axons). *Glial cell*s provide structural and physiological support for neurones and lie between blood vessels and neurone. About 90% of CNS cells are glial.

Nerve Fibres. These extensions of the cell body may be very long as in the case of those from motor neurones to the lower limb. Thicker axons become *myelinated*, that is, they acquire a wrapping of Schwann cell cytoplasm giving an insulating layer. (The Schwann cell is a special type of glial cell.) Thinner axons (the vast majority) remain nonmyelinated. The term nerve fibre is usually used to describe a myelinated axon.

Muscle Fibre-Type Grouping

Nerve damage may lead to loss of innervation to individual muscle fibres which will be re-innervated by adjacent nerve fibres ('collateral re-innervation'). This will lead to an increase in motor unit size resulting in loss of fine control. Conversion of the histochemical fibre-types will lead to fibre-type grouping.

Test Questions on Muscle & Nerve

1. Explain the following histological observation made in wax-embedded, H&E-stained sections.

   a) In smooth muscle cut in transverse section, not all profiles contain nuclei.

   b) White adipose tissue shows no sign of fat in a wax-embedded section

2. What do the blue granules in conventional sections of neurones represent?

[Answers at end of text]

LECTURE 4

BONE & BONE FORMATION

Bone is one of the three *Specialised Connective Tissues*. Rigid for weight-bearing. The matrix is largely composed of calcium salts (60% by weight). Collagen fibres are present. The cells are called *osteocytes*, and lie in lacunae which interconnect via narrow tunnels (*canaliculi*). Processes of the osteocytes extend throughout the canaliculi, which are continuous with the longitudinal, central [Haversian] canals and the radial, perforating [Volkmann's] canals, which carry blood vessels and nerves. The concentric layers or *lamellae* of matrix around a central canal form *osteons* [Haversian systems].

The inside and outside free surfaces of bone are covered by a layer of dense connective tissue, (*endosteum* and *periosteum*, respectively), which contains undifferentiated, pluripotent mesenchymal cells and [Sharpey's] collagen fibres.

Bone is not fixed, but is continuously being *remodelled* by organised processes of breakdown and formation of new osteons. The cells responsible for the resorption of bone are *osteoclasts*, which are giant cells with 200-300 nuclei, 15-20 of which may be visible in a single section. Osteoclasts are invariably found lying on the surface of the bone. Their cytoplasm is acidophilic (red with H&E) and highly vacuolated ('foamy') and they contain hydrolytic enzymes.

Bone may be classified as *spongy* or *dense*. Spongy (also known as 'cancellous') bone consists of a trabecular (lattice-like) structure, with many spaces between the strands. The strands of bone are covered by a thin layer of CT — *endosteum*. Dense (or 'compact') bone has no spaces within it. Compact bone is almost entirely composed of osteons; spongy bone may contain osteons; if it does not, it is known as 'woven bone'.

4.21 Bone as a Calcium Reserve. 99% of the calcium in the body is present in the skeleton — which therefore acts as a Ca^{2+} reservoir. Ca^{2+} may be mobilised by transfer of Ca^{2+} from newly-formed regions of bone to the interstitial fluid. Two hormones, *calcitonin* and *parathyroid hormone* (PTH) act on the osteoclasts to regulate the release of Ca^{2+} from bone. PTH is the principal regulator of plasma Ca^{2+} concentration and stimulates osteoclasts to increase bone breakdown and hence increase the release of calcium from bone. Calcitonin only acts when plasma Ca^{2+} is extremely high and inhibits the osteoclasts and reduces the mobilisation of calcium. [These hormones also act on renal handling of Ca^{2+}.] Lack of Ca^{2+} can lead to malformation or decalcification of the bones. Both vitamin D and vitamin A are required for the effective assimilation of Ca^{2+}.

4.22 Bone Formation. Bone is always formed by the conversion of an already existing tissue. Woven bone is formed first and then converted to lamellar (compact) bone.

The foetal skeleton is made of cartilage which forms the template for bone formation by *intracartilaginous ossification*. This is best seen in the epiphysis of a growing bone, where there are *two* processes occurring simultaneously: a) *growth in length*; b) *ossification*. It is these two processes that cause the characteristic zonation of growing bone. This zonation is the production of a dynamic process — the image we have is static. *[It is not necessary to remember the names of the zones but you should know what processes are occurring.]*

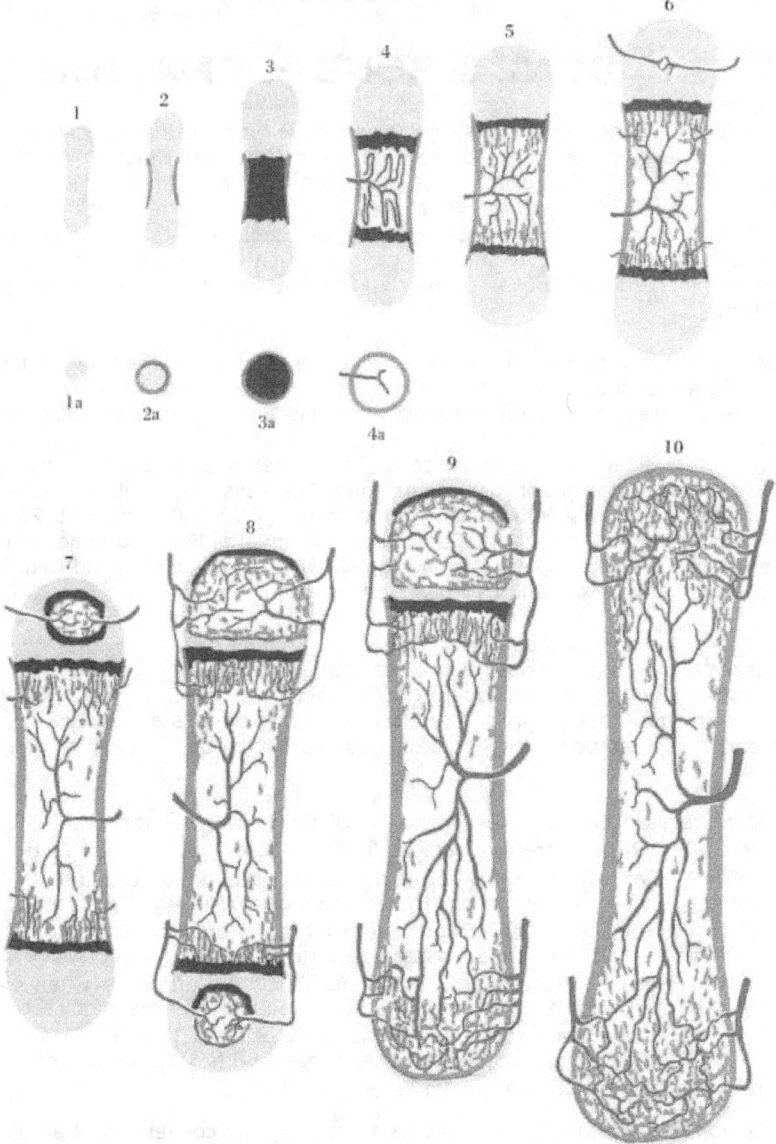

Figure 3. Bone formation (ossification).
The sequence proceeds from 1 to 10. Cartilage is represented by pale blue (eroding cartilage, dark blue), bone by pink; blood vessels by red).

    1)   is the cartilaginous model of the bone.
    2)   the bony periosteal collar forms.
    3)   Erosion of oldest cartilage.
    4)   Erosion forms the primary marrow cavity. Blood vessels and CT enter the primary marrow cavity.
    5)   The cavity enlarges rapidly. Erosion of the cartilage forms trabeculae.
  6-9) The secondary ossification centre is formed, resulting in the restriction of bone formation to the epiphyseal discs (as well as the sub-periosteum).
   10)   Eventually the epiphyseal disc is obliterated and no further growth can occur.

Summary of Bone Formation

a) *Growth in length* — occurs by the addition of new cartilage at the neck of the bone (*epiphysis*). At the extremity of the epiphysis the chondrocytes are small (Quiescent Zone), but towards the shaft (*diaphysis*) they are mitotic, forming columns of small cells (Proliferative Zone), which then increase in size (Maturation Zone).

b) *Ossification* (Fig. 3). Cells in the connective tissue sheath around the cartilage (*perichondrium*) differentiate into osteoblasts and form bone on the surface of the cartilage (the *periosteal collar* — pink in Fig. 3b). This process continues, adding to the growth of the bone.

At the same time, the chondrocytes in the middle of the shaft hypertrophy, the lacunae enlarge and the amount of matrix is correspondingly reduced and calcified (becoming basophilic) as in Fig. 3 (3). (In favourable circumstances it may be possible to see a 'tide-mark' of calcification where the matrix becomes basophilic — blue with H&E). The chondrocytes then die and the matrix is dissolved leaving only the thicker plates (*trabeculae*) like stalactites hanging down into the marrow cavity of the bone.

Blood vessels and cells grow into the spaces [Fig. 3 (4-5)] which are enlarged to form the *primary marrow cavity.* Some cells become osteoblasts and form bone on the remaining matrix — the whole constituting the *primary ossification centre.* This process extends outwards from the centre (Fig. 3 (5). The periosteal collar thickens to support the eroded cartilage.

Finally, bone is resorbed in the centre so that the thickness of the wall remains approximately constant while the overall diameter increases. The primary marrow cavity becomes filled with small precursor cells of blood and is therefore densely basophilic because their nuclei are so close together.

Thus, ossification forms four more zones (from end to middle): *Calcification, Retrogression* (death of chondroblasts and dissolution of matrix), *Ossification, Resorption*.

A *secondary ossification centre* develops at the epiphysis [Fig. 3(6)] and expands, leaving cartilage only on the articular surface and as a thin epiphyseal plate or disc. It is from the diaphyseal edge of this plate that further cartilage formation and growth occurs in childhood.

Growth in length of the bone ceases when the proliferation of the chondrocytes is not sufficient to keep pace with the rate of ossification and the epiphyseal disc becomes completely ossified.

––––––

Test Questions on Specialised Connective Tissues

1. Briefly describe the functions of the following cells: chondrocytes
    osteoclasts
    osteoblasts

2. Name the principal *processes* involved in bone formation.

3. What is the probable origin of the cells involved in fracture repair?

[Answers at end of text]

LECTURE 5

BODY FLUIDS

Objectives

a) To be able to describe the different fluid compartments of the body and outline the principles of their measurement.

b) To be able to state the approximate volumes of the major compartments of body water.

c) To be able to describe the movement of water and other molecules between compartments.

d) To be able to list the various forms of water input and output and state which are subject to physiological regulation.

e) To understand the role of plasma proteins in the movement of fluid across capillaries.

———

All cells are bathed in fluid and therefore depend for their functional integrity on the maintenance of the volume and composition of that fluid.

Definition of Compartments

Table of the Fluid compartments and their volumes, based on a normal, healthy, 70 kg male.

Compartment	Volume (litres)
Total Body Fluids (H_2O)	42
Intracellular Fluid (ICF)	28
Extracellular Fluid (ECF)	14
Plasma (Pl)	2.8
Interstitial Fluid (IF)	11.2

[After Sherwood, Fig. 12.2]

There are also Lymph and Transcellular compartments which are so small that they need not be considered in calculating the volumes of compartments. The Lymph compartment comprises the fluid passing to the plasma via lymph nodes. The Transcellular compartment comprises the fluid secreted by cells e.g. CSF, bile, urine etc.

Total body water accounts for 40 -80% of the body weight. Most of the variation between individuals is accounted for by variations in the amount of body fat — fat is only about 10% water.

Intracellular Fluid (ICF) is the water contained in the cells. The composition of each cell is separately regulated by intracellular mechanisms (ion pumps etc). Thus, different cells can have different compositions according to their functions. ICF is separated from the *Interstitial Fluid* by cell membranes.

Interstitial Fluid bathes all the cells and is the internal medium or *milieu intérieur* of Claude Bernard. Clearly, its maintenance is of critical importance to the function of the cells and hence the body as a whole.

Interstitial Fluid is one component of the *Extracellular Fluid* (ECF) and is separated from the *Plasma* by the walls of the blood vessels. There is a continuous *passive* interchange (osmosis, diffusion) between the Plasma and the Interstitial Fluid, so their compositions are very similar — with the notable exception of the Plasma proteins which cannot leave the blood vessels.

It follows that, if there is a large and rapid interchange, then if one compartment is regulated (volume and composition), the other is also regulated.

Comparison of ICF and ECF
There are important differences in composition because of the selective permeability of cell membranes (active and passive mechanisms) and the non-diffusibility of the intracellular proteins.

The principal differences are as follows.
  a) Specific non-diffusible proteins on both sides of the cell membrane.
  b) Na^+-K^+-ATP pump moves Na^+ out and K^+ into cells. Consequently, Na^+ is the predominate anion outside the cells and K^+ the predominant cation inside the cells. Cl^- follows Na^+ (so does $HCO3^-$).
  c) Inside the cells, the principal anions are $PO4^{3-}$ and Proteins (Pr^-) Intracellularly principal anions are $PO4^{3-}$ and Pr^-.

Osmotic Function of Plasma Proteins

The Plasma proteins are too large to leave the capillaries, and consequently provide an osmotic pressure tending to draw water into the capillaries from the interstitial fluid. This 'colloid osmotic pressure' (*oncotic pressure*) of about 25 mmHg is important in understanding the process of ultrafiltration and reabsorption of fluid in the capillaries, which is the essential mechanism of interchange between plasma and Interstitial Fluid. [Stanfield & Germann p 415 ff].

———————————————————————————————

———————————————————————————————

Arteriole Capillary BP   **Colloid OP**   **Capillary BP**
37 mmHg   **25 mmHg**   **17 mmHg**
Venule

———————————————————————————————

———————————————————————————————

NET OUTWARD PRESSURE   **NET INWARD PRESSURE**
~12 mmHg   **~8 mmHg**

Figure 4. Diagram to show Bulk Flow across the capillary wall. The osmotic pressure due to the Plasma Proteins (OP) [_oncotic pressure_] acts to draw fluid into the capillary. The blood pressure inside the capillary acts to force fluid _out_ of the capillary. Since the blood pressure varies over the length of the capillary, there is net _outward_ flow at the arteriolar end and net _inward_ flow at the venular end.

Significance of Bulk Flow.

The very permeable capillary wall allows plasma and solutes (not cells or proteins) to pass readily across (in both directions).This means that there is rapid interchange of materials between Plasma and IF. _BUT the composition (and volume) of plasma is carefully regulated (kidney); hence IF composition is carefully regulated._

Oedema [U.S. edema]

Oedema is the swelling of tissues following the accumulation of interstitial fluid. In the following summary of the causes of oedema, the above diagram should be used to work out the exact cause and effects. Oedema is important because it results in a reduced exchange between blood and cells and therefore the nutrition of the cells may be impaired. Note particularly the key role of the Plasma Proteins.

a) _Reduced Plasma Protein Concentration_ — results in reduced oncotic pressure and hence reduced absorption of interstitial fluid. Reduced plasma protein concentration can be caused by increased loss of proteins (e.g. renal disease or extensive burns); reduced protein synthesis (e.g. in liver disease); or dietary deficiency.

b) _Increased Capillary Permeability_ (e.g. after histamine release) — leads to leakage of Plasma Proteins in the interstitial fluid, with a reduction of the oncotic pressure and also a tendency to rein fluid in the interstitium.

c) _Increased Venous Pressure_ — causes increased capillary pressure tending to increase the outward flow of fluid from the capillaries. Occurs in congestive heart failure and in pregnancy when the uterus presses on the abdominal veins.

d) _Blockage of Lymph Vessels_ — impairs the normal removal of excess interstitial fluid. Occurs after removal of lymph nodes or parasitic infestation of lymph vessels (elephantiasis).

Both the composition (ions and proteins) and the volume must be kept within narrow limits to maintain normal body function.

'*Normal*' input is by ingestion and output via gut, urine, respiration and sweat. Of the outputs, only urine production can be regulated in relation to water balance.

In '*Abnormal*' or clinical and pathological situations there may be inputs via injection or infusion. Abnormal outputs are vomiting, diarrhoea, burns, haemorrhage. As an exercise consider whether water, salts, proteins or cells are lost or gained in each case.

The physiological responses to perturbations of fluid composition or volume are complex. For now, consider the general mechanisms of response to fluid loss.

Volume Regulation is by increasing intake of water (thirst centre etc.) and reducing the output of urine. The osmolarity of blood is monitored in the kidneys and the concentration of the urine adjusted accordingly.

Regulation of composition. Na^+ monitored in kidneys; erythrocyte levels monitored (see *Haemopoiesis*). In both cases appropriate physiological adjustments are made to counteract the deviation from normal values.

Test Questions on Body Fluids

1. What is the volume of Total Body Water in a normal, healthy 70 kg male?

2. What are the principal differences between intracellular water (ICF and extracellular water (ECF)? Explain these differences.

3. What is oedema and why does it occur in liver disease?

[Answers at end of text]

LECTURE 6

BLOOD I

Objectives (Blood)

a)   To be able to recognise, describe and classify the circulating blood cells and to briefly indicate their functions.
b)   To be able to outline the processes by which blood cells are formed.
c)   To be able outline the basis clotting mechanism and the role of platelets
d)   To be able to outline the fundamental mechanisms of anaemias.

Blood is a connective tissue. Its cells are dispersed in a liquid matrix (plasma); the fibrous component is 'latent', being produced only in the course of clotting. The cells occupy about 45% of the blood by volume (haematocrit).

It is important to be able to recognise all the circulating blood cells, because many of them migrate into the tissues and the different types present in pathological conditions are a fundamental diagnostic aid.

1. Histology of Blood Cells

Special stains (e.g. Wright's, Giemsa) are used to identify blood cells in smear preparations, because they show more detail than conventional histological stains, such as H&E. The pH reaction of these stains is the same as H&E; that is, acidophilic structures are stained red and basophilic structures are blue (see p 7). However, it is possible to identify many of the cells fairly reliably with conventional stains in sections by using the simple criteria of i) *size* and especially ii) *nuclear form*.

1.1 Erythrocytes (Red Blood Cells)
Small (mean diameter ~7 μm), no nucleus, pale centres due to biconcave shape. The cytoplasmic reaction is slightly acidophilic which means they appear pale red with the commonly-used stains. Erythrocytes are enormously common (5×10^6 /mm^3 i.e. 5×10^9/ml).

The lifespan of erythrocytes can be estimated by labelling with radio-active iron during formation (*'cohort labelling'*) and monitoring the disappearance of the label from the blood. The proportion of radio-labelled erythrocytes remains constant for several months then declines. The average life-span is about 120 days. (Clinically, the half-life is measured with chromium (*'random labelling'*) as 30d. This is an underestimate, due to loss of Cr; when corrected, the half-life is the expected 60d.)

Functions of Erythrocytes. The principal function is carriage of O_2 and CO_2, bound to haemoglobin (Hb). The biconcave shape of the cells aids diffusion by giving a large area and keeping the cell thin.

The cells are filled with Hb and have no organelles for synthesis or repair. Consequently their lifespan is limited. The cells are very flexible and can therefore pass through the smallest capillaries of around 3 µm diameter, As they age they become less flexible and cannot pass through the small capillaries and are usually removed by phagocytic cells in the spleen.

1.2 Leucocytes (White Blood Cells)

These are sub-divided into *granulocytes* and *agranulocytes*, according to the presence or absence of granules in the cytoplasm. Note that the granules are visible only with special stains). Leucocytes are rare (5-9 x 10^3/mm^3) compared to erythrocytes. A more detailed consideration of the functions of leucocytes is in *Blood II*).

Granulocytes (i.e. containing granules). Granulocytes are distinguished primarily by the staining reaction of their granules. It is important to assess the 'colour balance' of a particular preparation to assist in determining the staining reaction. Red blood cells are *slightly acidophilic,* and their staining reaction can be used as an inbuilt colour comparator, to determine the reaction of the granules of granulocytes.

Diagnosis of a particular cell type should be confirmed by the secondary criteria of *relative frequency* and *nuclear form.*

> *Neutrophils.* 70% of all leucocytes. The granules have a neutral reaction and are therefore paler than the slightly acidophilic red blood cells (rbc). In fact they may often be quite difficult to distinguish. There is a characteristic prominent, many-lobed nucleus (hence the alternative names of *polymorphonucleocyte* or *'polymorph.'* Motile and phagocytic. Lifespan approximately 60 hours. A high level of circulating neutrophils is associated with bacterial infection.

> *Eosinophils.* 2-4% of leucocytes. Granules redder (acidophilic) than the rbc. Nucleus bilobed. Lifespan 8-12 days. A high level of eosinophils is associated with parasitic infection.

> *Basophils.* Rare — less than 1% of leucocytes. The granules are large and coarse and almost always obscure the slightly-indented nucleus. The granules are basophilic (blue) and contain heparin and histamine. A high level of basophils is rare.

Agranulocytes (Lymphocytic cells). In both kinds of cell the nucleus fills most of the cell, leaving a thin rim of slightly basophilic cytoplasm. The lymphocytes and monocytes are associated with immune responses (see *Blood II*).

> *Lymphocytes.* Comprise 30% of leucocytes. Nucleus round or only slightly indented. Their size is variable but smaller than monocytes. Involved in immune responses.

> *Monocytes.* Comprise 5% of leucocytes. Their nuclei are indented or kidney-shaped. Becomes a macrophage after migrating into the tissues. They are the largest circulating blood cells. Involved in immune responses.

Platelets

Platelets are not cells but are fragments of the cytoplasm of large cells (megakaryocytes) in the bone marrow. Their frequency in blood is 25 x 10^3/mm^3. Platelets are concerned in the process of clotting. Lifespan 8-12 days.

2. Haemopoiesis

The continuous formation of the cells and platelets of the blood is necessary to keep their numbers relatively constant. In the human adult, blood cells are formed in certain bones (e.g. skull, ribs, sternum, ends of long bones). Before maturity, other sites are also involved (long bones, spleen etc.). The rate of production of blood cells is regulated by a complex hormone system.

It now seems most probable that all blood cells are derived from a single 'stem cell', the *haemocytoblast*, found only in the bone marrow. This stem cell has two possible fates. Its offspring may remain as stem cells, thus maintaining the pool of stem cells; or they may differentiate into one of the five specialised 'progenitor cells', each of can give rise to only one of the following cell types: erythrocytes, granulocytes, lymphocytes, monocytes or platelets (from megakaryocytes) (See Fig. 2). Each of these progenitor cells divides repeatedly ('amplification') to give a large number of descendants.

This is an example of the progressive restriction of a cell's potential; from a cell which can potentially form any one of the seven types of circulating cell, to a more restricted range of possibilities. Thus, after one division of a haemocytoblast, the daughter cells may be able to form any one of the three types of granulocyte (but none of the other cell types). After further division the daughters acquire granules specific to one cell type (e.g. a neutrophil) and that cell line is then restricted to that type.

Erythropoiesis. The formation of the red blood cells (rbcs), or erythrocytes, is taken as the example of haemopoiesis. The general pattern is the same for all cell types.

The *haemocytoblast* is the putative pluripotent stem cell capable of giving rise to all the circulating blood cells. There are only about 1-2 haemocytoblasts for every 1000 nucleated marrow cells. The haemocytoblast is large, spherical with basophilic cytoplasm and a round nucleus (i.e. relatively undifferentiated). In contrast, the erythrocyte is small (~8 μm diameter), common, without a nucleus, biconcave and slightly acidophilic due to the large concentration of haemoglobin (Hb).

The first recognisable stage in erythropoiesis is the *pro-normoblast* — a moderately large cell with a round nucleus filling most of the cell. The chromatin is dispersed; there are nucleoli, and the cytoplasm is basophilic.

The nucleoli disappear and the cell is now a *normoblast*. Several (divisions (3-5, forming 8-32 cells) over 5-7 days result in much smaller cells. Nuclei become shrunken and dense (pyknotic) and are extruded. Hb accumulates and makes the cytoplasm more acidophilic (pink with conventional stains).

Reticulocytes are formed when division has ended; they are still larger than rbc and with less Hb. They have a residual apparatus for synthesis of Hb. Reticulocytes continue making Hb and shrinking. They usually spend 1-2 d in the marrow before entering the circulation. Reticulocytes may be recognised after they have been released into circulation by staining for RNA.

Apply similar logic to all other cell types. The key point is the gradual restriction of potential and the acquisition of the features of the mature, circulating cell.

The following Table shows some normal haematological values. Note particularly the calculation of mean corpuscular Hb. You will have an opportunity to derive these values in laboratory classes.

	Male	Female	Units
Haemoglobin	13.6 - 16.9	11.6 - 15.8	g/dL
Haematocrit	43 - 49	36 - 45	%
MCHC	34	34	g/dL
Red Cell Count	5.4×10^{12}	4.8×10^{12}	/L
Mean Corpuscular Volume	87	87	fL
Mean Corpuscular Haemoglobin	29	29	pg
Reticulocyte Count	1.6 - 10.4	2.6 - 15.4	/1000 RBC

dL = decilitre (100 ml), fL = femtolitre (10^{-15} litre), pg = picogram (10^{-12} g)

————

Test Questions on Blood

1. For each cell type listed below give a clinical condition which would result in an increased numbers of those cells in the blood.
    a) neutrophils
    b) eosinophils

2. Give the function of the following cells: neutrophils, lymphocytes.

3. Name the cell type which is the precursor (ancestor) of all circulating blood cells.

4. In a conventional, wax-embedded section, which criterion for classifying circulating blood cells would be the most useful?

5. Given the concentration of erythrocytes in blood and that the total blood volume is (approximately) 5 litres, how many erythrocytes must be synthesised per *second*? [Only attempt this question if this type of calculation amuses you!]

[Answers at end of text]

BLOOD II — Immune System

Objectives (Immune System)

a) To be able to describe the origin and roles of macrophages and lymphocytes in immune function.
b) To be able to outline and distinguish innate and adaptive immunity.
c) To be able to describe the principal features of phagocytosis and inflammation.
e) to demonstrate a basic understanding of some immune disorders.

Role of the Immune System

Immune cells have the ability to differentiate between the cells of the body ('self') and other organisms ('non-self'). This is the key element in defending the body against pathogens such as parasites, viruses, bacteria and fungi. Damaged or mutant cells are also 'non-self' and are detected and removed.

Immune responses are very powerful and have harmful effects: allergies and autoimmune diseases (below). Hence immune responses contain self-limiting mechanisms (beyond the scope of this lecture, but see *Suppressor T cells* below).

Components of the Immune System

Leucocytes

The immune system consists of the white blood cells (leucocytes — see above) and the lymphoid tissues. All the white blood cells are produced in the bone marrow but the lymphocytes divide and differentiate in the lymphoid tissue, specialised tissue scattered throughout the body especially at the 'portals', such as the tonsils in the throat.

All the leucocytes are involved In immune responses but the most important are monocytes and lymphocytes. Recall that all leucocytes are essentially transitory in the blood and have their principal functions in the tissues.

Monocytes. In the tissues they are called *macrophages*. They have three main functions.
- ☐ Phagocytosis, engulfing and destroying pathogens, cell débris etc.
- ☐ Secreting signalling molecules (cytokines)
- ☐ Processing antigens and presenting them to lymphocytes

Lymphocytes. The two main functional types are *B cells* and *T cells*. B cells are derived from the bone marrow and clones in gut-associated lymphoid tissue (GALT) and produce antibodies to specific pathogens. T cells are derived from the thymus and destroy 'non-self' cells.

Recognition of 'Self' — depends upon *major histocompatibilty complexes* (MHC) which are carried on each nucleated cell and are peculiar to each individual (shared by identical twins). (MHC is not present on rbc.)

Immune Responses

There are two types of immunity: *Innate* and *Adaptive*. Innate is the body's natural defence system, irrespective of exposure to any pathogens. Adaptive mechanisms are developed in response to exposure to specific agents (pathogens, complex molecules etc).

Innate Immunity

Is non-specific, that is responds to the *first* exposure to any 'non-self' cell. This provides an *immediate* response while the slower, more specialised adaptive response is mobilised.

As well as the barriers to the entry of pathogens (skin and mucous membranes), the innate responses include phagocytosis, the inflammatory response and specialised chemical responses.

Chemical Responses

Interferon is produced by cells infected with *any* virus. It protects other cells against viral attack. In addition, it also slows cell division and enhances Natural Killer (NK) cells and cytotoxic T cells (below), properties which are used in cancer therapy.

Natural Killer cells attack any virus-infected cell, damage the cell membrane so that they to swell up and burst (lysis).

Note that both Interferon and NK cells will attack *any* virus-infected cell, so it is a non-specific response.

Complement System. This a class of molecules with many complex functions. The main function in the context of this course is recognition of micro-organisms and lysis (similar to NK cells). Reinforces many other inflammatory responses (hence the name!).

Phagocytosis. Both neutrophils and macrophages are phagocytic. 'Non-self' material is *attached* to the surface of the cell, taken into the cell (*internalised*) in a membrane-bound vesicle (phagosome). Lysosomes containing hydrolytic enzymes fuse with the phagosome and break down the contents (*degradation*). The remnants pass out of the cell by *exocytosis*.

Inflammatory Response. This is an extremely complex and powerful response and this course only outlines some of the basic processes. The 'aim' of the response is inactivate or destroy invading micro-organisms, remove the débris and prepare for healing processes. In favourable circumstances, normal function will be restored, but if tissue repair is incomplete, scar tissue may be formed with loss of function.

The initiating step is the release of *histamine* from mast cells ('tissue basophils'). Histamine has two effects on blood vessels: vasodilation, resulting in increased blood flow; increased permeability, allowing leucocytes and plasma proteins to enter the tissues. The leucocytes will begin phagocytosis etc. The proteins include complement, antibodies and clotting proteins (especially fibrinogen). The influx of proteins will cause oedema (see *Body Fluids*).

The characteristic symptoms of inflammation are *redness*, *swelling*, *tenderness* and *pain*. The first three are all accounted for by the influx of blood and the oedema. Pain is caused by local distension and mediating molecules released locally.

Adaptive Immunity

This is the response to specific agents which have been previously encountered. It is mediated by lymphocytes. B cells produce antibodies which circulate in the blood: a *humoral* or *antibody–mediated* response. T cells act directly on damaged cells— *cell-mediated* response. Both types of lymphocyte recognise foreign molecules (antigens) by means of antigen receptors on their surfaces. Each receptor binds only one antigen conferring *specificity*. However, there are millions of lymphocytes recognising millions of antigens so the system has *diversity*. Exposure to an antibody results in the production of clones of cells which recognise the specific antigen. *Memory* cells are long-lived so that another exposure to the antigen causes a rapid proliferation of the memory cells and large numbers of antibody molecules are produced in a few hours. (Recall that lymphocytes recognise 'self' and 'non-self' so the system has *self-tolerance*.)

Humoral/Antibody-Mediated Immunity. An antigen binds B cells and stimulates them to divide into *plasma cells* and *memory cells*. Plasma cells generate large amounts of the appropriate antibody. They are quite short-lived. The antibodies are secreted into the blood (hence 'humoral') as *immunoglobulins* (Ig). IgM and IgG are responsible for most immune responses. IgA is found in the secretions (saliva, mucus etc). IgE targets parasites. Memory cells persist indefinitely (see above).

Cell-Mediated Immunity. Antigen with MHC is required to activate T cells. Macrophages are the principal antigen-presenting cells. Division and differentiation of activated T cells gives rise to *cytotoxic T cell*, *helper T cells*, and *suppressor T cells*.

Cytotoxic T cells kill infected cells by lysis (see above). *Helper T cells* are about 70% of all T cells (see AIDS below) and are probably the key regulating cells of specific immune responses. They enhance the activity of cytotoxic T cells as well as phagocytic activity of macrophages etc. They also stimulate the development of B cells into plasma cells. *Suppressor T cells* secrete cytokines that suppress activity of B cells, as well as the above types of T cell. They also inhibit phagocytosis. This is one of the self-limiting mechanisms of the immune system.

Adaptive Immunity can also be *natural* or *artificial*, subdivided into *active* and *passive* mechanisms. *Natural immunity* arises actively by exposure to infection and passively by transfer of antibodies via the placenta or colostrum (first maternal milk). *Artificial immunity* arises actively by immunisation and passively by transfer of antibodies from another animal.

Immune Disorders

Autoimmune diseases — occur when the immune system fails to recognise 'self' and reacts against the normal tissues of the body. Examples are Systemic Lupus Erythematosus (SLE), Rheumatoid Arthritis (RA) and Multiple Sclerosis (MS).

Autoimmune Deficiency Disease Syndrome (AIDS) — caused by the human immunodeficiency virus (HIV) which specifically attacks Helper T cells, the key regulatory cells of the immune system. This leads to impaired immune function and hence increased susceptibility to infection, most notably pneumonia, TB and Kaposi's sarcoma. Infection of brain neurones leads to dementia.

———

Test Questions on Immune System

1. List the key features of innate and adaptive immunity

2. List the stages of phagocytosis.

3. List the characteristic symptoms of inflammation and explain each of them in terms of changes to blood vessels.

[Answers at end of text]

Answers to Test Questions

Epithelia
1. a) Number of layers of cells
   b) Shape of the *surface* cells
   c) Surface specialisation
2. *Squamous* — flattened; *cuboidal* — box-shaped; *columnar* — tall
3. Cilia, keratin

Connective Tissue Proper
1. Cells, fibres and matrix
2. a) The proportion of fibres (high — *Dense*; low — *Loose*)
   b) The arrangement of fibres (*Regular* or *Irregular*)
3. (b) White Adipose Tissue is pale in a conventional wax-embedded preparation because the fat is dissolved out by the alcohols used in the *dehydrating* stages.
4. By not dehydrating the tissue, e.g. by making *frozen* sections.

Specialised Connective Tissues
1. a) Chondrocytes produce and maintain the matrix of cartilage.
   b) Osteoclasts break down bone.
   c) Osteoblasts form new bone (initially on the cartilaginous trabeculae).
2. Elongation and ossification.
3. The connective tissues of the bone (periosteum, endosteum and invading vascular CT).

Muscle & Nerve
1.
   a) The cells are much longer than the nuclei; therefore many sections can be cut that do not include part of the nucleus.
   b) The fat is dissolved during dehydration.
2. Clusters of free ribosomes (RNA).

Body Fluids
1. 42 litres [NB *litres*, not kg or %]
2. Protein composition (proteins are largely non-diffusible)
   Na^+ is higher in ECF; K^+ lower (because of Na^+-K^+-ATP pump)
   [Important to understand that there is massive exchange between these two compartments.]
3. Oedema is the swelling caused by accumulation of excess interstitial fluid. In liver disease production of plasma proteins may be reduced leading to a reduction of the oncotic pressure and hence increased flow out of capillaries and decreased inward flow (see Fig. 4).

Blood
1. a) bacterial infection
   b) parasitic infection
2. Neutrophils — first line of defence in inflammation etc. Lymphocytes — immune responses
3. Haemocytoblast
4. Nuclear form
5. $\sim2.5 \times 10^6$

Immune System
1. *Innate*: non-specific, rel. rapid, first exposure to infective agent, phagocytosis, inflammatory response, interferon, complement

Adaptive: Specific, responds to later exposures, slower, lymphocytes(B humoral, T cell-mediated)

2. Attachment, Internalisation, Degradation, Exocytosis
3. Heat (increased blood flow— vasodilation), redness (increased blood flow — vasodilation), swelling (oedema due to protein leakage— more permeable vessels), pain (local distension, mediators)

www.ingramcontent.com/pod-product-compliance
Lightning Source LLC
Chambersburg PA
CBHW081244170526
45165CB00009B/3185